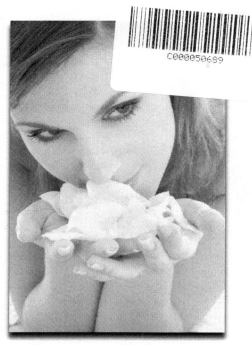

A DIY Guide to Therapeutic Body and Skin Care Recipes

Homemade Body Lotions, Skin Creams, Gels, Whipped Butters, Herbal Balms and Salves

(Art of the Bath Vol. 3)

Alynda Carroll

Ordinary Matters Publishing
P.O. Box 430577
Houston, TX 77243

www.OrdinaryMattersPublishing.com

A DIY Guide to Therapeutic Body and Skin Care Recipes
Homemade Body Lotions, Skin Creams, Whipped Butters, Herbal Balms and Salves

ISBN-13: 978-1-941303-08-5 (paperback)
ISBN-10: 1941303080
First Printing: October, 2014

Disclaimer and Terms of Use: Although the author and publisher have made every effort to ensure that the information in this book was correct at press time, the author and publisher to not assume and hereby disclaim any liability to any party for any loss, damage, or disruption caused by errors or omissions, whether such omissions result from negligence, accident, or any other cause. The author and the publisher do not warrant the accuracy of the information, text, and graphics contained within the book due to the rapidly changing nature of science, research, known and unknown facts, and the Internet. This book is presented solely for informational and entertainment purposes only.

Printed in the United States of America

Books by Alynda Carroll

The Art of the Bath Series

Custom Massage Therapy Oils
A DIY Guide to Therapeutic Recipes for Homemade Massage Oils

A DIY Guide to Therapeutic Bath Enhancements
Homemade Recipes for Bath Salts, Melts, Bombs & Scrubs

A DIY Guide to Therapeutic Body & Skin Care Recipes
Homemade Body Lotions, Skin Creams, Gels, Whipped Butters,
Herbal Balms and Salves

A DIY Guide to Therapeutic Spa Treatments
Homemade Recipes for the Face, Hands, Feet & Body

A DIY Guide to Therapeutic Body Butters
A Beginner's Guide to Homemade Body and Hair Butters

A DIY Guide to Therapeutic Natural Hair Care Recipes
A Beginner's Guide to Homemade Shampoos, Conditioners,
Rinses, Gels and Sprays

Life Hacks for Everyday Living Series

HOUSEHOLD HACKS
Super Simple Ways to Clean Your Home Effortlessly Using
Hydrogen Peroxide and Other Cleaning Secrets

Pick up your FREE report *Learn the Art of Self-Massage*:

http://www.ordinarymatterspublishing.com/massage-bonus

Praise for *The Art of the Bath* series

for *A DIY Guide to Therapeutic Spa Treatments from the Comfort of Your Home*

"Ahhhh this is a keeper! It's packed with awesome and easy to make spa like treatments. I love going to the spa, but in between spa treatments this book is as good as it gets. My favorites so far are the healthy coconut cuticle softener, the tension-relieving eucalyptus food massage oil treatment- so good oh and for a coffee junkie like me, the all-over coffee body scrub priceless! Great DIY spa treatments book."
~ Yvette (Amazon reviewer)

for *A DIY Guide to Therapeutic Bath Enhancements*

". . . easy to follow and very simple too. If you are looking for an book that you can easily follow and make you feel like a pro in no time when it comes to making soaps, bath salts and scrubs, this is the book to have!"
~ LH Thompson (Amazon reviewer)

for *Custom Massage Therapy Oils*

"As well as being relaxing, the benefits of massage can be physical as well as mental. This book is a great little guide to their therapeutic benefits, how to make your own massage oil and which blends are recommended to induce sleep, invigorate or enliven, boost the immune system and more. I will be taking the advice in this book on board, as I know how wonderful massage oils can be - it's just a case of knowing which ones are right to use, depending on the mood and/ or benefits you want to induce in the person receiving the massage." ~ Anna J (Amazon reviewer)

for *The Art of the Bath series*

"I love Carroll's DIY Bath series. They are all so welcoming and are full of all these great ideas. Must have." ~ Laura Pope (Amazon reviewer)

To my mother and grandmother,
true beauties in their own right.

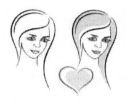

"Everything has its beauty, but not everyone sees it"

~ Confucius

.

A Note to the Reader

Perhaps, after relaxing in the bath and taking in all the benefits gained from a refreshing Art of the Bath ritual, you feel as though you are finished. Why wouldn't you? Maybe you spent some time giving yourself a self-massage with one of those custom blended massage oils you created. You have probably spent leisurely time luxuriating in a warm bath with your choice of bath enhancements such as bath salts, bombs, or melts. You may be feeling good, but you're not finished.

Smooth, soft, supple; as babies, we come into the world with skin designed to give and grow along with us. Eventually, though, inside and outside forces, such as hormones, lifestyle, aging, the sun's rays, and pollution take their toll, changing the quality and texture of our skin. The body and skin require attention.

Each year, cosmetic and pharmaceutical companies spend billions of dollars in an effort to develop products aimed at recapturing that baby-smooth skin softness. Unfortunately, these attempts often include unnatural ingredients. Instead, why not create your own products using natural ingredients to rejuvenate the skin?

This guide contains a collection of recipes that will help hydrate, soften, and restore the skin. The best time to use them is right after a bath when your body is most receptive. You'll find lotions, creams, gels, butters, salves, and balms that not only hydrate but also heal the skin. Why not extend that bath into a rejuvenating spa-like experience?

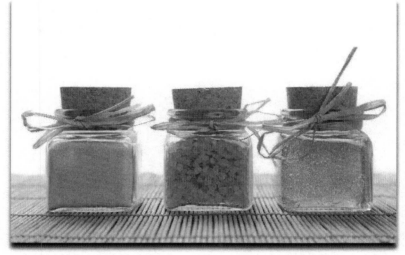

How to Give Yourself A Massage

Thank you for buying this book. In appreciation, I'm offering you this free report:

Learn the Art of Self-Massage

http://www.ordinarymatterspublishing.com/massage-bonus/

CONTENTS

INTRODUCTION

"Beauty is not the face; beauty is a light in the heart." —Kahlil Gibran

The idea of taking care of the skin is not new. Detailed writings go back to the time of the Ancient Egyptians describing beauty secrets and techniques, many often employed by royalty. Names such as Cleopatra and Nefertiti are attached to many ancient skin care techniques that are still in practice today. Ever hear of bathing in milk? You can thank the legendary Queen Cleopatra for that one. Queen Nefertiti was as entranced with cosmetics and their applications as any woman today.

With the skin being the largest organ of the body, it should come as no big surprise that we continue to be obsessed with its care. Our skin is our body's first line of defense against bacterial and environmental invaders. If we want to prevent or stall the ravages of daily life, then it's to our advantage to learn ways to keep our skin smooth and supple, free of cracks, scratches, or small openings that would allow those unfriendly forces entrance into our bodies.

There are any number of products you can create to keep the skin soft and healthy. Because the skin is clean and hydrated immediately after a bath that is the ideal time to apply skin care products. When we apply lotions and creams to our body, they are an addition to the skin's natural protective barrier, so less water is lost through evaporation, that is why our skin feels softer and smoother. As we age, our skin makes less of its own oil. Skin lotions and creams provide that needed additional support. Also, keep in mind that your face and scalp have an absorption rate that is ten times higher than other parts of the body. Performing a patch test is always a good idea, even more so if you have sensitive skin.

While the skin is a good barrier, some absorption does occur. That's why it's a good idea to use skin care products with beneficial natural or plant-based skin ingredients. A cream will sit on top of the skin longer than a lotion that will sink into the skin a matter of minutes. That said, absorption rates differ from person to person and ingredient to ingredient. One thing is certain, dry skin loves a good cream.

The various lotions, creams, balms, salves, and butters included here are not anywhere near as expensive as those you'll find at the beauty counters of your local department store. All you need is a kitchen, and you'll been on your way to making all-natural, therapeutic, after-bath products of your own.

While the recipes call for essential oils and speaks of their benefits. I am not a doctor or a scientist and have not performed any scientific tests on the ingredients. The ascribed benefits come from a long tradition of thought and use with these ingredients. In some cases, recent studies and research are confirming these beneficial attributes, but it's always wise to do your own research and testing, in this case skin testing, to make sure these ingredients are suited to you. Creating your own skin products is something that has been done thousands of years, and I am merely following in the footsteps and sharing what I've learned.

Now that we've covered all that, the time to begin is now.

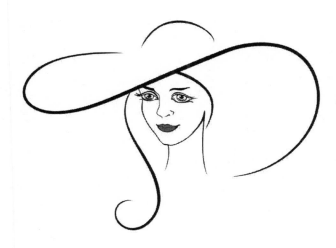

DIY Bath Therapy Products

Types of Skin Care Products

When was the last time you took a look at the skin care aisle of your local pharmacy? Do you remember how many types promised to restore and maintain your soft, supple skin? How do these products differ? Here's a short summary of their benefits:

Lotions – Lightweight and less viscous than a cream, lotions contain more water than creams and provide quick moisture absorption, usually through a pump dispenser.

Creams – Usually in jars, creams are thicker versions of lotions, containing more emollients to give them viscosity. They require more rubbing to be fully absorbed into the skin.

Gels – Gels are more concentrated than lotions, yet just as lightweight when applied. Ingredients may be added to provide the holding power necessary for hair styling products.

Whipped Body Butter – Whipped body butters are fluffier versions of creams. They contain all the moisturizing properties of a cream, but are effortless to apply.

Herbal Salves – Herbal-infused oils add healing ingredients to the protective properties of salves. Salves are meant to aid in pain relief, healing of scrapes or cuts, and in sealing a wound to protect it from germs and infection.

Balms – Balms also have the healing and protective qualities of salves. Where salves glide on the skin, balms are thicker and more lasting.

Getting Started

This collection of natural beauty recipes is for lotions, cream, gels, whipped body butters, salves, and balms. They are, by no means, the end-all but rather a starting point to get ready for your own explorations and creations.

Supply List

To get started you will need the following supplies:

Double Boiler – This is a small pot or jar in which to place ingredients, that is then put into a larger pot filled halfway with water. When the water in the large pot boils, it gently melts the ingredients in the smaller pot or jar, ensuring the mixture will not burn.

Wooden spoons or skewers for stirring. It is not advised to use metal utensils, since the metal may chemically react to some essential oils.

Measuring cup and spoons

Tongs – To prevent becoming burned from handling hot jars.

Grater – For grating beeswax into small pieces for quicker melting.

Funnel or spouted measuring cup – For pouring lotions into dispensers.

Containers – Whether the products are for personal use or as gifts, there are several ways to package your products. These include: mason jars, breath mint tins, decorative jars or vessels, or tubes and dispensers sold especially for these kinds of products. Whichever container you use, make sure it has an airtight lid.

SAFETY FIRST!

While essential oils are derived from natural products, that doesn't mean that you may not have side effects or reactions. If there is any doubt about how you will react to any of the ingredients in these recipes, it is wise to test a small amount on your skin before using. Also, although these products are made of natural ingredients, you should never ingest them.

Essential oils are the volatile aroma compounds from plants, and are potentially hazardous. They can cause irritation, allergic reaction, or become toxic with extended use. It is recommended that pregnant woman and children NOT be exposed to essential oils. Again, before you start a recipe, make sure the ingredient works for you.

Chamomile

An example is chamomile. While chamomile oil has wonderful benefits, for those who are allergic to ragweed, this oil may not be a good choice. The chamomile is in the ragweed family. Also, someone with sensitive skin may want to test oils like peppermint and wintergreen to make sure they either don't have a reaction. In some cases, less is best. However, with those who are truly sensitive, caution might suggest that you use an alternative oil.

Wintergreen

Wintergreen has a reputation for helping with arthritis and many other health problems, but caution is needed. Wintergreen has analgesic properties, and should therefore not be taken by anyone who has problems with aspirin or aspirin-like products. It is also suggested that anyone who is taking blood-thinning medications not use Wintergreen. You should definitely read up on this and other oils to make sure you know whether it is appropriate oil for you and your needs.

Beauty Lotion Recipes

LIGHT AND FRESH ROSE-LAVENDER MOISTURE LOTION

The calming effects of lavender and the uplifting properties of rose combine to create a lotion that is moisturizing as well as edifying. This is a perfect lotion for the days when the skin feels dry. The gentleness of the apricot kernel oil adds even more nourishment. Benzoin is an oil that has long been used not only for its fragrant long-lasting vanilla-like scent, but its ability to help the skin's elasticity as with its use in lip balm.

Ingredients:
1/4 cup + 2 tbsp Rose water
1/4 + 2 tbsp glycerin
1 cup Apricot Kernel oil
1/2 cup Beeswax
1/4 tsp Tincture of Benzoin*
2 drops Lavender essential oil

Directions:
In a measuring cup or small bowl, combine rose water and glycerin thoroughly. Set aside. In a small pan, place oil and wax, and then place pan in a larger pan that is filled about halfway with water. Melt over medium heat. Stir well. Once melted, remove from heat, and add the rose water and glycerin mixture, stirring well until cool. Add Benzoin and Lavender essential oil. Stir well and pour into desired container.

Store up to nine months.

*Benzoin should not be used by pregnant women or those who have sensitive skin or are prone to rashes.

PICK-ME-UP SPORTS SOOTHING LOTION

This warming lotion is the perfect anecdote for sore or aching muscles. Peppermint and eucalyptus essential oils are especially revitalizing after a good workout. Combine the two and you have the perfect after-sports pick-me-up.

Ingredients:

1/2 cup Sweet Almond oil
1/4 cup Coconut oil
1/4 cup Beeswax
1/4 cup Shea butter
1 teaspoon Vitamin E oil
2 drops Peppermint essential oil
2 drops Eucalyptus essential oil

Directions:

In a small pot or jar, place all ingredients. Next, place the pot into a larger pot that's been filled about halfway with water. Melt all ingredients, except essential oils, over medium heat, stirring well. Once ingredients are melted, cool slightly before adding essential oils. Pour the liquid into your desired container. Let cool completely before attaching lid. Apply generously to aching muscles and work in until warm.

Store for up to six months.

LEMON LIFT BODY LOTION

This is a wonderful, extra-moisturizing lotion that makes everything better. The lemon will instantly improve your mood, and the coconut oil will provide extra hydrating and valuable anti-oxidants.

Makes approximately 6 ounces of lotion.

Ingredients:
1/2 cup Coconut oil
1 tbsp Beeswax
10 drops Lemon essential oil
2 tbsp Distilled Water

Directions:
Grate beeswax until there is 1 tablespoon and place it in a small pot or jar. Add coconut oil, and place pan or jar into another larger pan that's halfway filled with water. Melt ingredients over medium heat, stirring often to thoroughly combine. Once melted, add lemon essential oil. Remove from heat and cool for 10 minutes. After cooling, pour ingredients into a blender, adding up to 2 tablespoons of water, and pulse mixture until it becomes the texture of thin pudding and is able to be dispensed through a pump dispenser. Pour lotion in into pump container

Store in cool, dark place for best results.

Skin Cream Recipes

SIMPLE UNSCENTED BODY CREAM

For those who want a simple, unscented cream, this is a winner. Maybe you're sensitive to scents, or perhaps you don't want to wear too many competing scents. Whatever your reason, you'll find this simple body cream to be a great addition to your skin care war chest. This thick body cream has the extra-rich moisturizing qualities of olive oil and coconut oil combined with the healing properties of beeswax and Vitamin E that makes for a terrific nourishing combination.

Ingredients:
1/2 cup Olive oil
1/4 cup Coconut oil
1/4 cup Beeswax
1 tsp Vitamin E oil

Directions:
Place ingredients in a small pan or jar. Pour water into a larger pan or pot to about halfway. Place the smaller pan, with ingredients, into the larger pot. Cook over medium heat until ingredients melt. Stir often to combine ingredients. Once fully melted and combined, pour the mixture from the small pan into the container you wish to use. (Not intended for pump bottles). Let stand until liquid becomes solid. and cools completely before attaching lid.

Store for up to six months.

ALMOND-HONEY MOISTURIZING BODY CREAM

If you live in a hot, humid climate, you'll love this cream. The addition of honey to this cream creates a richer texture with the extra nutrients honey offers. Honey is also a great humectant so the skin retains moisture. Great for those who have dry or itchy skin.

Ingredients:
1/2 cup Sweet Almond oil
1/4 cup Coconut oil
1/4 cup Beeswax
1 tsp Vitamin E oil
1 tsp Organic Honey
2 tsp Almond extract

Directions:
Place ingredients in a small pan or jar. Pour water into a larger pan or pot to about halfway. Place the smaller pan, with ingredients, into the larger pot. Cook over medium heat until ingredients melt. Stir often to combine ingredients. Once fully melted, add almond extract and combine. Pour the mixture from the small pan into the container you wish to use. (Not intended for pump bottles). Let stand until liquid becomes solid and cools completely before attaching lid.

Store for up to six months.

GRAPEFRUIT REJUVENATING BODY CREAM

The uplifting, citrus scent of grapefruit combines well with extra emollient benefits of coconut, olive, and Vitamin E oils to create a cream that both rejuvenates the skin and reinvigorates the spirit. To change things up a bit, you might want to try a different oil like eucalyptus. Grapefruit oil is often recommended for those with oily skin.

Ingredients:
1/2 cup Olive oil
1/4 cup Coconut oil
1/4 cup Beeswax
1 tsp Vitamin E oil
15 drops Grapefruit essential oil*

Directions:
Place ingredients in a small pan or jar. Pour water into a larger pan or pot to about halfway. Place the smaller pan, with ingredients, into the larger pot. Cook over medium heat until ingredients melt. Stir often to combine ingredients. Once fully melted, remove from heat, add grapefruit essential oil, and combine. Pour the mixture from the small pan into the container you wish to use. (Not intended for pump bottles). Let stand until liquid becomes solid and cools completely before attaching lid.

Store for up to six months.

*Those with sensitive skins may have a reaction to grapefruit oil. Do a test before using this oil in any recipes. Grapefruit oil may also increase sensitivity to ultraviolet light, so use a sun block if you're going to spend any time in the sun.

Gel Recipes

CLASSIC SIMPLE ALOE VERA GEL

Aloe Vera has a long history touting the benefits of this plant when applied to the skin. Aloe Vera is pretty much a staple around our house due to its many beneficial uses. This is a great gel to have on hand during hot summer months when the risk of sunburn is high. You can also use this gel to help soothe cuts from shaving or small scrapes or burns, apply this soothing Aloe Vera gel after bathing.

Ingredients:
Aloe Vera plant
500 mg Vitamin C tablet (crushed)
400 IU Vitamin E gel cap

Directions:
Slice outer layer of an Aloe Vera leaf. Peel away skin. Scoop out the gel and place in a measuring cup. Continue doing this with other leaves until there is ¼ cup of aloe gel. Put gel into a blender and add crushed Vitamin C tablet. Cut open Vitamin E gel cap and pour oil into blender. Blend all ingredients together. Pour into sterilized glass jar.

Store in the refrigerator for up to four months.

APPLE FIRMING NECK GEL

We often focus on the face and forget the neck. This recipe is great to help firm and smooth the neck as well as the face. Use this gel after bathing. You'll probably have enough of the mixture left for one more use.

Ingredients:
4 tsp Distilled water
1 tsp Apple juice (freshly juiced)
1 tsp 100% Pure Aloe Vera gel
4 tsp Vegetable glycerin
1 tsp Powdered pectin

Directions:
Heat water. Combine hot water, juice and Aloe Vera gel. Add glycerin to mixture and stir well. While liquid is still warm, add pectin. Blend with hand mixer to completely dissolve pectin. Set aside for up to half an hour or until mixtures becomes a light gel.

Apply gel to clean, damp neck. Leave on for 15 minutes. Rinse with warm water, pat dry.

Store in the refrigerator for up to a week.

FRAGRANT JASMINE HAIR GEL

Jasmine is a common oil used in hair care products because of its many benefits. Scalp massages are enhanced with the use of jasmine due to increased blood circulation. Many report how jasmine nourishes hair and helps those with dry and frizzy hair. In addition to the light fragrance, this gel is made without alcohol or chemicals.

Ingredients:
1/4 tsp Unflavored Gelatin
1/2 cup Distilled Water
6 drops Jasmine essential oil

Directions:
Heat water. Put gelatin in a small bowl. Add hot water to gelatin and mix well until the gelatin is completely dissolved. Refrigerate for 3 hours. Once mixture has set, add essential oil, and stir to combine. Using a funnel, place mixture into small squeeze bottle. Apply to damp hair and style.

Store in refrigerator for up to two weeks.

Whipped Body Butter Recipes

YLANG YLANG SWEET WHIPPED BODY BUTTER

Ylang Ylang has many health benefits and is known to help keep the skin in balance and hydrated. The light and lovely floral scent provides a romantic back note for the emollient properties of the Shea butter and the coconut and almond oils.

Ingredients:
1 cup Shea Butter
1/2 cup Coconut oil
1/2 cup Sweet Almond oil
10-30 drops Ylang Ylang

Directions:
Place all ingredients, except essential oils, in a pan. Place that pan into a larger pan that's been filled about halfway with water. Put both pans over medium heat and melt ingredients, stirring often to combine well. Once ingredients are melted, remove from heat and cool slightly before adding essential oils. Start with a lower amount of the Ylang Ylang oil and work your way up to the higher number of drops. Place in the refrigerator until the mixture begins to harden. Remove from refrigerator and mix with a hand mixer until fluffy. Place in desired container and return to refrigerator for about 10 minutes for mixture to set.

Store for up to nine months.

TANGERINE-WINTERGREEN WHIPPED BODY BUTTER

Wintergreen is refreshing and tangerine is cheerful. What better way to compliment a bath than by finishing it off with these two happy scents and skin smoothing cocoa butter. In addition, tangerine oil is often used in skin care products due to its ability to help refine the texture of skin. Wintergreen is often used in skin care products when relief is needed for sore muscles due to its analgesic qualities.

Ingredients:
1 cup Cocoa Butter
1/2 cup Coconut oil
1/2 cup Jojoba oil
10 drops Tangerine essential oil
10 drops Wintergreen essential oil*

Directions:
In a double boiler (a pan within a larger pan filled halfway with water), melt the butter, coconut oil and jojoba oil over medium heat. Stir as ingredients melt to combine thoroughly. Once melted, remove from heat and allow cooling slightly. Add essential oils until desired scent strength is achieved. Stir well and refrigerate until mixture is almost hard. Remove from refrigerator and whip with a hand mixer until fluffy. Place in desired container and then back in refrigerator for approximately 10 minutes for mixture to set. Remove from refrigerator and attach lid tightly.

Store for up to nine months.

*While wintergreen oil is a common essential oil, you should still make sure that it is the right oil for you. Due to its aspirin-like qualities, it is not recommended for those who need to avoid aspirin or aspirin-like products. In addition, this oil should not be used if you are on blood-thinning medication. Do not leave wintergreen oil around children or babies as it is toxic if ingested.

EASY COCONUT WHIPPED BODY BUTTER

Coconut oil is regularly touted for its many health benefits. The enriching oil is a wonderful ingredient for the skin, too. Coconut oil melts into your skin to nourish and nurture. Sun-parched skin will guzzle this rich emollient and the coconut scent will tease and conjure tropical retreats.

Ingredients:
1 cup Cocoa Butter
1/2 cup Coconut oil
1/2 cup Olive oil
1 tsp Vitamin E oil
20 drops Coconut essential oil

Directions:
In a double boiler (a pan within a larger pan half-filled with water), melt the butter and first three oils over medium heat. Stir as ingredients melt, to combine thoroughly. Once melted, remove from heat, and allow cooling slightly. Add essential oil until desired scent strength is achieved. Stir well, and refrigerate until mixture is almost hard. Remove from refrigerator, and whip with a hand mixer until fluffy. Place in desired container and then back in refrigerator for approximately 10 minutes for mixture to set. Remove from refrigerator, and attach lid tightly.

Store for up to nine months.

Herbal Salve Recipes

PLAIN OLD COMFREY SALVE

Comfrey is well known among herbalists for its traditional role in healing bone, skin, and muscle and is especially therapeutic for healing wounds or skin problems. I like to keep comfrey slave on hand all the time. Be sure you thoroughly clean wounds or skin areas before you apply this salve as it is known to promote quick healing and could heal the tissue on top of a wound while the dirt and bacteria remains inside and results in an abscess. The solution: Clean the wound first.

Ingredients:
2 oz. Dried Comfrey leaves
4 oz. Extra Virgin Olive oil
3/4 oz. Beeswax
10 drops Camphor essential oil

Directions:
In a small pan or glass jar, place the olive oil and dried Comfrey leaves. Place this pan into a larger pan filled halfway with water. Over medium-low heat, simmer for 3 hours. Place a strainer over a small bowl, and then cover strainer with cheesecloth. Pout oil and herb mixture into the cheesecloth to strain. Squeeze all the oil through the cheesecloth until it is completely captured in the bowl. Discard herbs.

Place Comfrey-infused oil and grated beeswax into a small pan and then place into larger that's filled halfway with water. Melt ingredients over medium heat. Stir well to combine. After ingredients have liquefied, remove from heat and add essential oil. Pour into sterilized jar or tin.

Store in cool, dark location for up to a year.

COMMON CALENDULA SALVE

The Calendula is a flower that many around the world turn to it for its skin healing abilities. You may know Calendula by its more common name: the pot marigold. Those with sensitive skin respond well to this salve. Many use Calendula Salve for a variety of conditions including chapped lips, dry skin, minor burns, and rashes, particular diaper rash. (You can also add a few drops of lavender essential oil, too.)

Ingredients:
2 oz. Dried Calendula
4 oz. Extra Virgin Olive oil
3/4 oz. Beeswax

Directions:
In a small pan or glass jar, place the olive oil and dried Calendula. Place this pan into a larger pan filled halfway with water. Over medium-low heat, simmer for 3 hours. Place a strainer over a small bowl, and then cover strainer with cheesecloth. Pour oil and herb mixture into the cheesecloth to strain. Squeeze all the oil through the cheesecloth until it is completely captured in the bowl. Discard herbs.

In a double boiler (a pan within a larger pan filled halfway with water), melt over medium heat Calendula oil and beeswax. As melting occurs, stir until well combined. Once melted, remove from heat, and pour into sterilized jars or tins.

Store in a cool, dark place for up to a year.

ARNICA PAIN RELIEVING SUPER SALVE

Arnica is an effective pain reliever for aching muscles and joints. I first learned of arnica's healing properties from a local pharmacist when I suffered a really bad sprained ankle and can testify to its ability to reduce swelling. The addition of Marjoram essential oil adds anti-inflammatory properties to the salve.

Ingredients
1 cup Extra Virgin Olive oil
1 oz. Dried Arnica
1/2 oz. Beeswax
1/4 tsp Vitamin E
1/2 tsp Marjoram essential oil

Directions:
In a small pan or glass jar, place the olive oil and dried Arnica. Place this pan into a larger pan filled halfway with water. Over medium-low heat, simmer for 3 hours. Place a strainer over a small bowl, and then cover strainer with cheesecloth. Pour oil and herb mixture into the cheesecloth to strain. Squeeze all the oil through the cheesecloth until it is completely captured in the bowl. Discard herbs.

Pour oil back into its original small pan (reserving a small amount in case it's needed later). Place smaller pan into larger pan. Add beeswax to the oil and additional water to larger pan (if needed). Over medium heat, melt the beeswax, stirring often to combine with the oil. Test for firmness by placing a tiny amount on wax paper and cooling in the refrigerator. For firmer salve, add more beeswax. If not firm enough, add more oil.

Remove from heat and add vitamin E and essential oil. Mix well. Pour mixture into container or tin. Let cool completely and attach lid.

Store in cool, dark place for up to one year.

Balm Recipes

A TIGER OF A BALM

Tiger Balm is a commercial product that is often considered a staple for the medicine chest. The balm is used for sore muscles and even headaches. This is a similar recipe. Unlike Tiger Balm, this balm adds spearmint for its uplifting qualities and to help revitalize those tired muscles. The cinnamon oil causes the warming effect of the balm. Those of you who have sensitive skin may need to reduce the amount of cinnamon oil. If you do have sensitive skin, make sure you do a patch test before using these ingredients.

Ingredients:
2 oz. beeswax
1/2 cup Olive oil
20 drops Spearmint essential oil
20 drops Camphor essential oil
8 drops Clove essential oil
10 drops Cinnamon essential oil

Directions:
In a double boiler (pan within a larger pan filled halfway with water), melt over medium heat the beeswax and olive oil. Stir as melting occurs to blend thoroughly. Remove from heat and stir in essential oils, adding until desired fragrance strength is obtained. Pour into small jar or tin, and close lid immediately. Cool before using.

Store for up to one year.

HEFTY MUSCLE BALM

Lavender is often used in rubs and balms for its medicinal qualities. Lavender is a great aromatherapy oil and is often added to recipes as a natural muscle relaxer for sore muscle strains. Many who suffer from muscle spasms, injuries, pain, and fatigue look to lavender for relief. Next time you have a Charley Horse, you'll be glad you whipped up this recipe, and after a hard workout or a long day you'll be rubbing this balm into your muscles for immediate relief. Remember, lavender oil is also used by many for its sedative effects, so consider the amount you add when creating your balm, as it may strengthen the effects of any medication you may be taking.

Ingredients:
1/2 cup Coconut oil
3 tbsp Beeswax pastilles
2 tbsp Shea butter
1/2 tsp Vitamin E oil
20 drops Lavender essential oil

Directions:
Melt ingredients in a double boiler (pan within a larger pan filled halfway with water), over medium heat. Stir ingredients to combine well while mixture melts. Remove from heat, and add lavender essential oil. Pour into desired container and attach lid. Cool well before using.

Store for up to six months.

PEPPERMINT TINGLE LIP BALM

Lip balm is simple to make and cost-effective. If you like to use lip balm to keep your lips hydrated, or you need to use a balm of some kind because your lips chap easily, this is a great recipe for you. You'll love the way the way the peppermint oil adds a quick pick-up as it refreshes your lips.

Yields 5 tubes of lip balm

Ingredients:

2 tsp Coconut oil
2 1/4 tsp. Beeswax
2 1/4 tsp. Sweet almond oil
1/3 tsp. Olive oil
1 tsp. Peppermint extract

Directions:

Melt all ingredients, except extract, in a double boiler (a pan with a larger pan filled halfway with water) over medium heat. Stir well to thoroughly mix all ingredients. Remove from heat, and stir in peppermint extract. Pour mixture into small tubes or tins, and let harden.

Conclusion

Sorry to say we're at the end of this collection. I hope you've enjoyed reading through the contents and have been inspired to start your own collection of natural skin care products. There are so many essential oils, and I've only touched on a few basic ones to get your started. Don't be afraid to play and develop your own ideas based on your needs. Our skin always needs attention.

Let's face it, biological, lifestyle, and environmental factors take a toll on your skin every day. As we age the skin becomes drier. What we eat, drink, and do plays an important part in our skin's overall health. Environmental elements, such as smog and dangerous UV rays, can change the texture and elasticity of the skin. It's impossible to avoid this daily assault.

As I've mentioned before, the good news is that we can create skin care products that will revitalize and rejuvenate the skin. Applying them immediately after the bath provides the best way to combat all these daily skin stressors. All these lotions, creams, gels, butters, balms, and salves are as accessible as your own garden and pantry. The effort is minimal, and the reward is great.

Not only is it fun to create your own skin care products, it's also a pretty thrifty way to pamper yourself.

I'm deeply thankful that you have taken the time out of your day to read through these pages. I hope you've enjoyed your time, and that you will continue on to enjoy and nourish your body with these wonderful all-natural recipes. Be sure and look for my other books that relate to the whole "art of the bath" experience.

Alynda Carroll

PS: I hope you've enjoyed this book and will take a few minutes to leave a review. Reviews are a big help for authors as well as readers.

About the Author

Alynda Carroll has loved baths since she was a little girl. Bubble baths, lotions, and creams have fascinated her. She spent many hours watching her mom create homemade beauty recipes. Later, Alynda's interests expanded to include herbs, essential oils, aromatherapy and the art of the bath as it is today.

Be sure and buy the rest of Alynda Carroll's best-selling books that make up her popular series The Art of the Bath, s well as her new series Life Hacks for Everyday Living. Look for the excerpt from her new book HOUSEHOLD HACKS at the back of this book.

MORE BOOKS BY ALYNDA CARROLL

The Art of the Bath Series

Custom Massage Therapy Oils: A DIY Guide to Therapeutic Recipes for Homemade Massage Oils

A DIY Guide to Therapeutic Bath Enhancements: Homemade Recipes for Bath Salts, Melts, Bombs & Scrubs

A DIY Guide to Therapeutic Body & Skin Care Recipes: Homemade Body Lotions, Skin Creams, Gels, Whipped Butters, Herbal Balms & Salves

A DIY Guide to Therapeutic Spa Treatments: Homemade Recipes for the Face, Hands, Feet & Body

A DIY Guide to Therapeutic Body Butters: A Beginner's Guide to Homemade Body and Hair Butters

A DIY Guide to Therapeutic Natural Hair Care Recipes: A Beginner's Guide to Homemade Shampoos, Conditioners, Rinses, Gels and Sprays

Life Hacks for Everyday Living

HOUSEHOLD HACKS: Super Simple Ways to Clean Your Home Effortlessly Using Hydrogen Peroxide and Other Cleaning Secrets

ALYNDA CARROLL

What's New?

Turn the page to read an excerpt from HOUSEHOLD HACKS. To receive updates on the release of Alynda Carroll's next books in the Art of the Bath series and BEAUTY HACKS, go to:

www.SimpleLivingHacks.com

Excerpt from
HOUSEHOLD HACKS

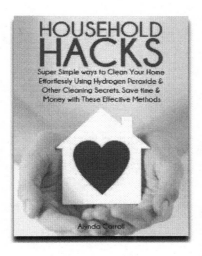

Welcome to Household Hacks, my personal collection of more than 200 cleaning tips, tricks, and household hacks for all areas of the home with an emphasis on using natural, inexpensive cleaners and strategies. Many have been around for a long time, but others are focused on the way we live today.

The advantages are many. You'll save money, time, and energy. You'll also become more effective at housecleaning by using these tips and strategies that will free up your time.

You'll find information about well-seasoned natural cleaners that have been helping people clean for generations and understand why they are gaining popularity today.

You'll discover cleaning strategies and hacks for various rooms including the kitchen, bathroom, and bedroom, as well as the home office. You'll even find creative living hacks to make home life easier.

This collection captures my favorites and includes additional hints and alternatives. If you already have a deep interest in DIY household hacks and natural cleaners, you will probably come across some familiar cleaning remedies. They will serve as reminders, but be of more interest to readers who are just starting down this more natural and simplified way of living. However, newer strategies and ideas will encourage you on your own journey toward living a more natural, clean, and simple life.

A major plus about having this book is that everything is gathered in this one place. This is a good, fun, and definitely useful reference to have on hand.

How the Book is Organized

The book begins by taking a look at the top natural cleaners in use today. There are several cleaning hacks and tips for each cleaner. I like to have a list of things I can do with a particular cleaner, as well as a collection of cleaning tips particular to an area of the home. The second section offers additional cleaning suggestions and creative household hacks for the kitchen, bathroom, bedroom, laundry and closet, living room, home office, and, by extension, the car.

- ❑ Natural Cleaners
- ❑ Hydrogen Peroxide
- ❑ Vinegar
- ❑ Baking Soda
- ❑ Lemon and lemon juice
- ❑ Apple Cider Vinegar
- ❑ Salt
- ❑ Household Hacks
- ❑ Office and Technology
- ❑ Bathroom
- ❑ Kitchen
- ❑ Bedroom
- ❑ Laundry and Closet
- ❑ Car
- ❑ Creative Hacks

Now that you have an idea of what *HOUSEHOLD HACKS* contains, are you ready to discover its treasures?

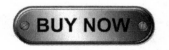

Buy your copy of *HOUSEHOLD HACKS* today.
www.SimpleLivingHacks.com

NOTES

INDEX

Made in the USA
San Bernardino, CA
16 October 2017